I0830923

HOUSEHOLD REMEDIES AGAINST SHINGLES

The 38 Best Household Remedies Against Shingles

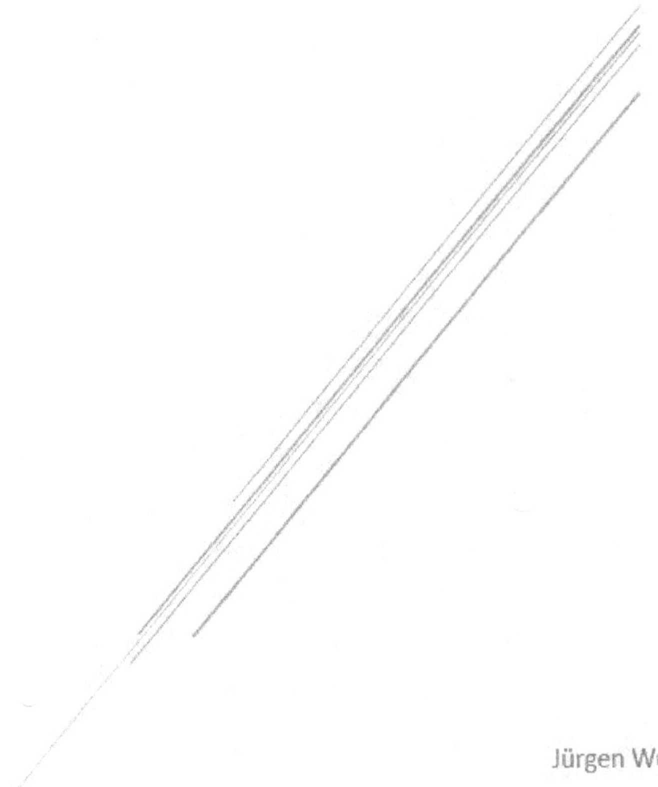

Jürgen Wude

Imprint

Contents

What is shingles?

Shingles is actually a secondary illness that can develop after contracting the chickenpox virus. In many cases, this illness does not occur until decades after the initial infection with the virus.

Shingles is a very painful and unpleasant skin rash that usually appears on one side of the body and is characterized by its belt-like appearance. It is caused by the varicella-zoster virus (chickenpox virus), which belongs to the genus of the herpes viruses. The varicella-zoster virus can trigger two different disease patterns: chickenpox and shingles (herpes zoster).

In most cases, the virus triggers the dreaded childhood disease chickenpox first. Until the vaccination was introduced, most of those who were affected usually experienced the illness in childhood. Unlike the chickenpox rash, which disappears again after you overcome it, the varicella-zoster virus stays in your body. Similar to other herpes viruses, this virus invades both the nerve roots of the spinal cord as well as the cranial nerves and remains in the human organism for a lifetime.

In the event of an outbreak, the formerly dormant viruses travel to the skin surface via the nerves and shingles develop. All areas of the body, including the face or the brain as well as various organs, can be affected.

How does shingles develop?

The viruses remain inactive in the human body for decades until they are finally awakened and the disease breaks out. The triggers can vary greatly: Advanced age, extreme stress, other diseases or a weakened immune system can all cause shingles.

There is often no clear reason why the viruses break out again. Mainly elderly people are affected, as their immune system becomes weaker with increasing age than in younger years. It is possible for young adults and children to suffer from shingles, but this happens very rarely.

The most frequent causes of shingles are:

- Extreme stress, for example great emotional distress.
- UV radiation: Excessive UV exposure can trigger shingles, for instance after a severe sunburn.
- Any kind of infection, even a mild flu infection, can favor the occurrence of shingles.
- AIDS: The HI virus destroys important cells of the immune system and weakens it.
- Cancer diseases often negatively affect the immune system.
- Chemotherapy: Fighting cancer also results in a weakening of the immune cells.
- All medication that dampens the functioning of the body's immune system (immunosuppressants), for instance in a rheumatism therapy with TNF blockers.
- Congenital defects of the immune system.

Who can develop shingles?

Only people who have already been infected with the varicella-zoster virus, which causes shingles, can suffer from the disease. The first infection usually takes place during childhood. Whoever has fallen ill with chickenpox once could also suffer from shingles later on.

But people who are vaccinated against chickenpox can generally also have shingles. However, they fall ill with the malicious disease far less often and the disease progression is normally markedly weaker. In these cases, the rash typically appears where the vaccine injection occurred.

How long does the disease last?

The duration of the disease can vary. Decisive factors are the affected individual's general state of health and physical constitution. If the immune system is severely weakened, the disease can also last longer, for the body's defense system needs more time to successfully fight the viruses. Patients who have a strong immune system oftentimes experience a significantly shorter disease duration, as their defense system can control the viruses more quickly.

The time of treatment is also crucial for the disease duration and the disease progression. If shingles is identified at an early stage and is treated in a targeted manner, the duration of the disease is usually shorter.

Yet, the disease duration can be prolonged if shingles is not recognized right away and the therapy begins at a later point. If this is the case, the disease progression can be far more severe. In addition, there is a higher probability of permanent damage and complications.

Therefore, a herpes zoster infection should be treated as soon as possible, ideally two to three days after the first symptoms appear. The age of those affected also has an influence on the duration of the disease. Elderly people often suffer from shingles for a longer period of time compared to younger ones.

The first erythemas appear within three days after the viruses have been reactivated and can also be accompanied by pain. What follows is an unpleasant neuralgia of the nerve cords that have been infected with the virus. After about three to five days, the blisters that are typical of the disease begin to appear on the skin.

Around five to seven days after the viruses have been reactivated, the blisters pop open and small, open wounds develop. They eventually heal and the characteristic scabs form on the skin. The duration of the incrustations depends on the severeness of the shingles. When all of the blisters have popped and the wounds are crusted, the disease is no longer contagious.

If shingles is treated properly, it heals completely within two to four weeks. If the course of the disease is particularly severe, however, complications can occur and a follow-up treatment may be necessary. Moreover, this can also lead to consequential damages. It is not uncommon for those affected to suffer from the typical neuralgia even long after they have shingles.

How do I recognize shingles?

The first sign of shingles is experiencing pain in a certain skin area, which is accompanied by a slight fever and weariness. Particularly the torso is frequently affected. At first, the affected skin area is reddened until the characteristic blisters that can be unpleasantly itchy finally appear. After a few days, the blisters pop open and begin to encrust.

Shingles can be very dangerous, it can also affect the face or especially the eyes (zoster ophthalmicus). If it develops in the optic nerve, the cornea or the iris, it may even result in blindness. If shingles occurs in the ears (zoster oticus), the facial nerve can become inflamed, which causes a facial paralysis.

In rare cases, shingles can also lead to meningitis or an inflammation of the brain. If the immune system is significantly weakened, shingles can also extend to several parts of the body and cause life-threatening complications.

Is shingles contagious?

The virus infectivity is very high, which means that there is also a high risk of infection. Tests have shown that 90 out of 100 test persons contracted chickenpox if they had had direct contact with an infected person. Every person who has not had chickenpox yet can generally infect others.

If a person has shingles, direct contact with others should be avoided. For the varicella-zoster viruses can be transmitted through contact with the blisters on the skin or their virus-containing substance. This can happen if a healthy person comes into contact with the infectious skin rash of an affected person.

Moreover, you can also get shingles if you touch objects that an affected individual previously held in their hands. However, if you have not been vaccinated or have not had chickenpox, you contract chickenpox first, not shingles. It is not possible to suffer from shingles right away, it can only break out later, if the viruses remaining in the nerve cells are reactivated for any reason.

By the way: Chickenpox can not only be transmitted through direct contact, but also by droplet infection. This can even happen if a person encounters a sick individual who is several meters away.

The reason for this is that the pathogen can be passed on very quickly through the air and the respiratory system. A single virus-containing drop is enough to infect a patient with chickenpox. This is also why very many people can contract the virus at large gatherings at once.

Treating shingles

Traditional medical practice predominantly uses pain killers and antiviral medication to treat shingles. Moreover, it is also very important to pay attention to careful skin care.

Paying attention to thorough skin care and treating the rash in a targeted manner constitute central aspects when treating a herpes zoster infection (shingles). In order to prevent additional bacteria from infecting the affected skin areas, corresponding powders are often used.

In addition, drying, itch-relieving and antiseptic gels and lotions can bring relief. Important active ingredients are menthol, zinc, podicanol as well as tannins. If blisters have already formed, those suffering from shingles can perceive moist and cooling compresses to be very pleasant. The compresses can also help against the bad itching and terrible pain.

Pain killers are usually used to alleviate acute pain. If you have slight pain, acetylsalicylic acid (ASA) or paracetamol can suffice. Affected persons can buy compounds like these without a prescription at a pharmacy. If shingles is accompanied by fever, these medications can also lower the fever.

If you are suffering from severe pain, it is often necessary to use strong pain killers. In this case, school medicine often turns to opioids such as tramadol, which, however, are only available on prescription and can have side effects.

The trigger of shingles – the varicella-zoster virus – is combatted directly with antiviral agents. These drugs are called virostatics and they ensure that a replication of the viruses is inhibited. Typical antiviral agents are for example valaciclovir, brivudine or aciclovir.

If the disease is treated with antiviral medication, the duration of the pain can be shortened and the healing accelerated. A precondition is always that the therapy is begun as soon as possible. Virostatics are usually taken in tablet form, but if the disease is particularly severe, the treating doctor can also administer infusions.

Treating shingles with virostatics is generally reasonable, but it is not absolutely necessary in every case. Especially with young patients or cases where there is no severe form of the herpes zoster infection and no complications are to be expected, antiviral agents do not necessarily have to be used.

The situation is different for those suffering from a severe illness and risk patients, like individuals who are more than 50 years old or have a weakened immune system. The same goes for cases where shingles appear on the head, the neck or the face, or if the course of the disease is particularly severe.

A typical characteristic of shingles is a stripe-type rash on the chest or also on the back. The unpleasant blisters, which are accompanied by an irritating itchiness and strong pain, are also typical of the disease.

A vaccination can also prevent the outbreak of shingles if you have not had chickenpox yet. Therefore, it is recommended that children and young people get a vaccination.

What is treacherous and dangerous is that 70 % of those affected continue to suffer from neuralgia even after shingles has disappeared. Greatest care must be taken if shingles appears on the head or the face. The viruses can affect the eyes and cause conjunctivitis or a corneal inflammation. Moreover, this can lead to damages of the optic nerve or diseases like glaucoma. Even the ear can be affected, whereby possible consequences are an impaired balance, facial paralysis or a sudden hearing loss.

In addition, it can also be risky if pregnant women suffer from shingles. The unborn child is protected during pregnancy, but the baby can be infected during birth. Aside from a herpes zoster infection, this can also lead to other serious diseases.

Shingles can also be treated with household remedies. Particularly in cases where conventional medical treatments do not help, an alternative therapy with proven household remedies is an option.

Moreover, household remedies can also be an excellent addition when treating shingles with a therapy based on traditional conventional medicine. Many of these remedies against shingles are always within reach in every household. Therefore, affected individuals can react to the disease particularly quickly and promptly counteract the symptoms with household remedies.

Household remedies against shingles

Compress with cold milk

The skin rash that accompanies a herpes zoster infection can be extremely unpleasant, very itchy and can also hurt. Cold milk is ideal to calm the inflamed skin, which is why a compress with cold milk is a recommendable option. For this purpose, a towel or a washcloth is soaked in cool milk and then loosely wrapped around the affected skin areas.

Milk contains a lot of vitamin A, vitamin C and calcium. The nutrients in milk can strengthen the upper layer of the skin (epidermis), reduce the undesired skin reactions and support the regeneration of the skin. Affected individuals can easily use a compress with cold milk several times a day.

Ice compress

An ice compress can also be very soothing to alleviate the symptoms of shingles. The ice can cool and calm the irritated skin and effectively reduce the itchiness and pain. Additionally, the coldness increases the blood circulation, stimulates the skin's metabolism and can therefore support the revitalization of the skin.

However, the ice should not be in direct contact with the inflamed skin, for if the ice is too cold, it can cause frostbite. Therefore, it is beneficial to use an ice compress. For this purpose, ice cubes are wrapped in a towel and placed on the irritated skin. This compress can be used as long as the ice cools the skin.

If necessary, an ice compress can be applied several times a day to reduce the symptoms. Added to this, the compress can also be used to alleviate the pain after the blisters have popped open and during the healing process.

Baking powder and water paste

Baking powder is a true all-rounder. It can be helpful for various ailments and problems and is a practical helper you should always have at home.

If you mix it with water, it becomes a paste that is also known to be a proven home remedy to treat shingles. To make the paste, simply stir baking powder into some water until it becomes a firm, but still spreadable mush.

Afterwards, the baking powder and water paste is applied right to the inflamed skin or the blisters. The paste dries out the blisters, which can soothe the inflammation and cause the entire rash to subside. In addition, it can significantly reduce both the itching and the pain.

Vinegar and honey paste

The itching sensation can also be alleviated with a vinegar and honey paste. It should be carefully applied to all of the affected skin areas. Aside from drying out the blisters, the paste can also reduce the inflammation of the skin.

With more than 90 valuable ingredients, apple vinegar can be especially good for skin health. Natural vinegar is pH-neutral and can strengthen the acid mantle of the skin. The skin is provided with several important nutrients such as beta-carotene, folic acid, bioflavonoids or vitamin C that can refresh and revitalize it. In particular, this can have a positive effect on wound healing.

Honey has anti-inflammatory, disinfecting and antibacterial properties. By using honey, the inflammation of the skin that accompanies shingles can be alleviated. In addition, further and advanced skin infections as well as a spreading of the herpes zoster infection can be prevented.

Thanks to the many positive characteristics of vinegar and honey, a combination in the form of a paste proves to be ideal to treat shingles.

Medicinal herb cat's claw

Cat's claw is an ancient medicinal herb used by American Indians. In Peru, the herb has been used to treat various ailments for several centuries. Its positive effect on viral diseases has also been proven by recent scientific studies. The cat's claw root (Radix Uncariae tomentosae) is used for therapeutic application.

In the fight against the herpes zoster infection, the body's immune system and metabolism play a particularly important role. This is where the medicinal herb cat's claw can help, for the natural remedy is attributed with a strengthening effect on the immune system and the metabolism.

Aside from its antiviral characteristics, cat's claw also has anticarcinogenic, antioxidant and anti-inflammatory properties. Therefore, the medicinal herb can be used specifically to alleviate the inflammatory rash.

In Austria, cat's claw can be bought in pharmacies without prescription. In Germany, the medicinal herb is often part of dietary supplements. Cat's claw can be taken in capsule form or as a tea.

It is important to drink lots of liquids when you are suffering from a viral disease, ideally a kind of tea that can promote the healing process. Especially melissa tea has proven effective in the fight against shingles, for melissa has an antiviral effect. If you have shingles, you can drink two to three cups of the tea a day. Once it has cooled down, melissa tea can also be applied directly to the infected skin areas to reduce suffering. For this purpose, any commercially available kinds of melissa tea can be used. What is important is to prepare the tea according to the instructions.

Melissa tea can also be made with melissa leaves and used for external application afterwards. For this purpose, roughly 150 ml of boiling water are poured over about 6 teaspoons of melissa leaves. The tea should brew for approx. 10 minutes. Then, a cotton cloth is soaked in the tea and you can use it to gently dab the affected skin areas.

By the way: Melissa can not only have a calming effect on the body, but also on the mind.

It is also known that green tea has numerous health-promoting properties. Green tea can be used to fight and prevent bacteria and viruses particularly due to its high content of certain antioxidants. These antioxidants (EGCG) can prevent viruses from attacking the healthy cells and using them as a host.

This way, the growth and spread of viruses can be prevented and existing infections can be alleviated. The tea can already unfold its full effect when only small quantities are used. Therefore, drinking around half a liter of green tea a day can help reduce the discomfort caused by shingles.

Tea made from fenugreek, melissa, juniper and oats can also have a pain-relieving effect. It is prepared by combining 10 g each of the four ingredients. Afterwards, you pour 250 ml of boiling water over the mixture. The tea should brew for 15 minutes before it is drunk hot.

Water and epsomite paste

If you are suffering from shingles, the body's self-healing powers can also be supported with a simple paste made of water and epsomite. This paste has both an anti-inflammatory and a drying effect and can be prepared very quickly without much effort. You simply stir epsomite into water until it becomes a spreadable mixture. This paste can be applied to the inflamed skin areas several times a day, which can keep the inflammation at bay and reduce itchiness.

Moreover, the blisters can be dried out with the water and epsomite paste, with the effect that the skin can heal better and more quickly. Additionally, it can prevent the rash from spreading and ensure that it goes away more quickly. The paste can also lower the risk of further infections through other bacteria, which can find an ideal breeding ground in the rash and the open wounds.

St. John's wort or linseed oil

Linseed oil can also contribute to the healing of shingles. You simply apply it right to the affected skin areas that itch or hurt. The blisters can also be treated with linseed oil in a targeted manner.

In ancient Greece, people swore by the positive effects of linseed oil, which can score particularly with its very high content of Omega-3 fatty acids. The oil can promote our general health, strengthen the cardiovascular system in particular and thus help the body tackle the viruses and symptoms.

St. John's wort oil is one of the most well-known natural remedies for nerve diseases. If this oil is applied to the inflamed skin, it can be very soothing for those suffering from shingles, as the pain can be noticeably relieved. If you do not want to apply St. John's wort oil right on your skin, you can soak a cloth with it and place it on your skin. The oil can be bought at several pharmacies, drugstores and health food stores.

A lukewarm compress with the tannin-containing medicinal herb oak bark can also support the healing process during the final stage of shingles. For this purpose, a cloth is soaked in an oak bark decoction and the compress is wrapped around the infected parts of the body. The decoction can support wound healing and help reduce the infection.

Oak bark decoction can be bought at some pharmacies and health food stores, but as an alternative, you can also make it yourself. Simply mix 100 grams of oak bark with around a liter of water and bring it to a boil in a pot.

After about 20 minutes, the oak bark decoction is ready. Then, you strain the decoction and let it cool down before the compress can be made. By the way, the oak bark decoction can also be used for a relaxing and soothing bath by adding the same amount to the bathing water.

The tannins that oak bark contains, around 28 %, make it so valuable for those who are combatting shingles or several other illnesses. These tannins – among them catechin, epicatechin, ellagitannins as well as complex tannins – can strengthen the skin. Oak bark has an astringent effect on the skin, which means that it is more difficult for bacteria to enter it, and at the same time, it can also have a positive impact on the itchiness.

When applied externally, oak bark should generally be used for a maximum of two to three weeks on a regular basis. If you use it too often, damage to the liver can occur.

If the rash hurts and itches a lot, the skin can also be treated with 100 % pure aloe vera gel. The gel cools the skin and can calm it. At the same time, it can counteract an unpleasant drying out of the skin and keep the symptoms from getting worse. It is important to use 100 % pure aloe vera gel without any additional scents.

Today, we know more than 300 different aloe vera plant types. However, only three of them have been proven to have a health benefit. In nature, the plant only grows in desert areas with a tropical climate. But aloe vera can also flourish in your home as a pot plant.

Aloe vera is used both in agriculture and in medicine. In addition, it is a highly decorative plant. Aloe vera is an important ingredient in many products such as cosmetics, lotions, ointments or also drinks.

The plant has been used as a remedy since around 3000 before Christ. Indigenous peoples have employed it for various medical purposes. Aloe vera is attributed with a very positive effect on skin problems. The ancient Egyptians even mentioned the plant in their holy writings more than 5000 years ago.

Aloe vera juice can be used as an alternative or a supplement to the plant's gel, as it is a proven home remedy that can put a stop to the almost unbearable itching caused by shingles.

In order to obtain 100 % pure aloe vera juice, the plant is simply cut into small pieces so the juice can run out. Then, the juice is carefully spread on the itching and hurting skin areas. When used externally, aloe vera juice has an optimum effect on inflammations.

You can also drink the juice, which has a distinctive bitter taste. Aloe vera contains more than 200 different active ingredients. If you drink its juice or apply it externally, the human body can be ideally supplied with nutrients.

What is special about aloe vera is not only the amount of active ingredients, but also the unique combination of the individual components, which enables them to ideally unfold their full effect.

Of course, aloe vera juice is not a miracle cure, but it can be beneficial for the body in many ways. Above all, this unique plant can support the metabolism and ensure that toxins and harmful substances are eliminated.

In addition, drinking aloe vera juice or applying it to your body can prevent possible deficiency symptoms. But what is especially important is that it strengthens the body's immune and defense system. This helps the body cope with the herpes zoster infection.

No matter whether white cabbage or kale, cabbage is a home remedy that has been known for centuries. Thanks to its many antioxidants, it can help ease the symptoms of various illnesses, including shingles. The cabbage leaves can alleviate the rash in the form of a poultice or a compress.

Cabbage can contribute to an improvement of the skin cell structure. Its leaves contain a lot of moisture, which is why it can prevent the skin from drying out. Using cabbage leaves can also reduce the risk of scar formation.

In alternative medicine, the medical plant cabbage is often employed to support wound healing. This also applies to shingles, as the burning rash can be significantly reduced with cabbage leaves. Particularly white cabbage contains many anti-inflammatory active ingredients. The inflammatory stimulus can be weakened considerably if the cabbage leaves come into contact with the purulent blisters.

Many of those affected report that they are overcome with a noticeable relief and confirm that the irritating and tight skin sensation in the concerned body areas can disappear completely. For cabbage also creates a cooling effect, as the medical plant has a very high water content. Even if cabbage leaves are cut up, they still release a lot of moisture.

Cabbage leaves calm skin areas that are plagued by shingles. In this context, it is also beneficial that cabbage contains B vitamins, which have a positive influence on the nerve fibers. White cabbage can convince with the B vitamins B1, B2, B6 and B12.

A cabbage poultice can easily be made with cabbage leaves, you only need fresh, juicy white cabbage. Aside from the mentioned active ingredients, white cabbage also offers a wide range of ingredients, particularly with vitamin B, potassium and calcium, in the fight against shingles.

The cabbage leaves should be thoroughly washed under running water before they are used. For in the worst case, dirt or residues of germs could increase the existing rash, lead to other undesired skin reactions or trigger further infections through bacteria.

Large cabbage leaves are especially suitable for a compress. First, the large leaves are carefully separated from the cabbage and the wide leaf vein is removed. In order for the ingredients to unfold their full effect, the cabbage leaves should be cooked in a water bath. Once they are cooked, it is necessary to let the cabbage leaves cool off. Then, the leaves are carefully dabbed and squeezed with a kitchen towel so they can dry. Afterwards, the cabbage leaves can be placed right on the inflamed parts of the skin. It is important to do this gently, to prevent the blisters from accidentally bursting open. Otherwise, the herpes zoster viruses could spread to other areas of the skin.

Cabbage leaf poultices can remain on the skin for several hours. To fix them, you can use a cotton cloth or you could even wrap a loose gauze bandage around them, if necessary. This cabbage poultice can be used repeatedly until the rash subsides.

In most cases, there is a noticeable alleviation of pain after only a few days. Moreover, the cabbage leaves can cause the pustules to dry out and disappear more quickly. However, the typical, unpleasant smell of cabbage leaves takes some getting used to.

If you have a herpes zoster infection, you should make sure to pay attention to a corresponding nutrition. Foods containing capsaicin, such as chili peppers, should definitely be on the menu, as spicy food can ease the suffering. Capsaicin can help against neuralgia. In addition, foods containing capsaicin can also contribute to alleviating the itching caused by the rash. Capsaicin can be found in nearly all kinds of peppers and in cayenne pepper.

Due to the activation of the TRPV1 receptor, capsaicin generally relieves pain. The receptor is overstimulated and finally becomes insensitive to other stimuli. As this receptor is responsible for making us feel pain stimuli, it is possible to reduce the pain this way. The receptor also transmits heat signals and is part of the reason why we can taste pungency.

Various vitamins and minerals can strengthen the immune system, reduce the pain caused by shingles and generally be effective against the herpes zoster infection. In this context, a combination of vitamin B complex with vitamin C and vitamin E can be particularly effective.

B vitamins can alleviate pain and support the nervous system. For instance, B vitamins are important for the development of the so-called myelin layer, which is the protective layer of individual nerve fibers. By taking a vitamin B complex, the nerves can be protected during a herpes zoster infection. B vitamins play an important role in the functioning of the human nervous system. Not only can they reduce neuralgia, but they can also control inflammatory reactions and optimize the effect of painkillers. It is assumed that B vitamins unfold their pain-relieving effect in various ways. For instance, vitamins B1, B12 and B 6 can contribute to the recovery and renewal of damaged and injured nerve fibers. In addition, they can improve the ability to transmit individual nerve signals.

Particularly vitamin B12 has been attributed with an extremely positive effect on the disease process of shingles, although corresponding long-term studies are still lacking. Nevertheless, it is useful to take vitamin B12 when you are suffering from shingles. As the various B vitamins are closely connected with each other in the human body and carry out many processes together, it is always advisable to consume a vitamin B complex.

In order to alleviate the pain you experience when you have shingles, it is recommended to take up to 500 mg of vitamin B12 in the form of methylcobalamin. The exact dosage should be approved by the treating physician. People who have shingles and are also suffering from a kidney disease are only allowed to take vitamin B12 as methylcobalamin, for if it is taken in the form of cyanocobalamin, it can damage the kidneys.

When you take vitamin C, the pain can be reduced. There are many indications suggesting that vitamin C has a pain-relieving effect, though this mechanism has not been fully resolved yet. However, it is known that vitamin C belongs to the most effective antioxidants and can protect both tissues and cells from damage resulting from oxidative stress. In addition, it exhibits anti-inflammatory properties that can also have a positive impact on pain relief. Vitamin C also positively influences the immune system, with the result that the likelihood of contracting viral infections is lowered.

A lack of vitamin C can be identified as a risk factor for arising pain as well as post-zoster neuralgia. For compared to healthy people, individuals who are affected by post-zoster neuralgia have rather low vitamin C levels or a vitamin C deficiency. If you are suffering from post-zoster neuralgia, vitamin C is oftentimes administered as an infusion to quickly alleviate the symptoms.

Experts recommend supplying your body with around 1000 to 2000 mg of vitamin C per day to strengthen the immune system. It is advisable to take vitamin C in several small doses over the course of the day. The vitamin is very well tolerated if you take it with food.

Vitamin E comprises a group of similar compounds, namely Tocopherols, which can have an antioxidative effect. This vitamin is essential in the fight against free radicals, in order to prevent cell damage.

Similar to vitamins A, K and D, vitamin E is a fat-soluble vitamin. It can only be absorbed via the lipid metabolism. Therefore, a dietary intake is only possible if the body is simultaneously supplied with some fat. Alpha-tocopherol is the best-known vitamin E.

The valuable cell protection vitamin can diminish the inflammatory reactions that occur when you are ill with shingles. Moreover, a good vitamin E balance can increase the skin's resistance, inhibit inflammations and improve wound regeneration. The daily requirement depends on sex, age and several other factors. Vitamin E can especially be found in vegetable oils such as sunflower oil, wheat germ oil, thistle oil or rapeseed oil, but it can also be absorbed via food supplements.

Avoiding agitation and stress

Too much excitement, enormous stress and emotional distress can severely weaken the immune system. Various stress factors can make the body react to certain challenges or demands in a natural, but unspecified way. Your breathing becomes faster, your blood pressure increases, your heart rate rises and your muscles tighten. It is a mere survival reaction of the body that is based on evolution. In addition, this leads to an increased release of stress hormones and the body produces additional energy. This scenario repeats itself every time a condition that is perceived to be dangerous, uncontrollable or stressful arises.

Various things can be responsible for this, such as exam nerves, problems in your partnership or in the family, trouble at work, traumatic experiences, serious illnesses, bad accidents or fear of the future. The problem in today's world is that the body is running on full speed, while the additional energy is not reduced like it used to be in the past. If these or other forms of stress continually arise, this creates a permanent stress situation and negative stress builds up. This permanent negative stress often triggers the malicious illness shingles. It is extremely likely that negative stress can even be an immediate cause of shingles, while the varicella-zoster viruses rather play the role of the indirect cause of the viral disease.

If stress leads to an activation of the viruses in the organism, there are different signs that can help you detected this early on. Among these signs are an unexpected inefficiency, frequent tiredness and a permanent weariness, hurting or heavy limbs, fever, flu symptoms as well as a burning sensation, itching or even a numbness in the nerves. If these indications are recognized, those affected should immediately try to avoid negative stress. For the typical, very unpleasant rash or shingles itself only appears when a nerve path is completely inflamed. Therefore, a timely reduction of stress can prevent the outbreak of shingles. At the same time, it can be helpful to start treating the smoldering shingles as soon as first signs are detected.

If you want to prevent shingles, you should try to avoid permanent negative stress. The methods for this are mostly individual. First, the stress factors need to be identified. Once this has taken place, they should be eliminated, which frequently goes hand in hand with a change in the usual lifestyle habits. As this is not always immediately possible, outlets can also help relieve negative stress and excess energy, for example by doing yoga, physical exercise or taking a vacation.

Compress with olive leaf extract

Olive leaf extract is one of the most effective home remedies against numerous different pathogens due to its many valuable substances and especially due to the antioxidant oleuropein as well as its high content of elenolic acid. It is also successfully used in particular against the herpes zoster virus. Olive leaf extract is employed to treat the flu, candida infections or, as already mentioned, shingles. What is more, the extract can not only render harmless pathogens, but also support the regeneration of the inflamed skin areas.

To treat shingles, it is advisable to use a compress with olive oil extract. To make the compress, immerse a cotton cloth in olive leaf extract and place it on the affected body areas for some time. The itching skin blisters can already disappear after only a few days. At the same time, olive leaf extract can also prevent scarring. Moreover, it can be taken in capsule form in addition to the compress, whereby the capsules' oleuropein content should be at least 15 to 20 % for an optimum effect.

Calendula salve

If shingles is already well advanced and the skin blisters have burst open and are scabbed, typical ailments like itchiness and tightened skin can be treated externally with calendula salve. The salve can increase the healing process and prevent strong scarring.

Due to its good skin tolerance and the broad spectrum of efficacy, calendula salve should not be missing in any medicine cabinet. The salve can have an antibacterial, wound-healing, decongestant and anti-inflammatory effect. The reason why calendula salve is so effective has to do with its contents that include flavonoids, essential oils, coumarins and saponins, all of which can be found in the plant's blossoms.

Moreover, calendula salve can also be used after the acute phase of the illness, for the post-treatment of the skin or scars. Provided that those affected do not have an allergic reaction to composite plants, the salve can be employed without any problems, for there are no known side effects.

Affected areas should be extensively and generously treated with calendula salve. It is advisable to gently massage in the salve in circling motions because this ensures that its substances can ideally be absorbed by the skin.

In order for the skin rash to disappear as quickly as possible and all of the other symptoms to be alleviated as well, it is useful to treat the affected areas of the body with the calendula salve several times a day. The healing process can also be supported by letting the skin areas get a lot of air. You can make the salve yourself or find it at a pharmacy.

Magnesium

Magnesium can play an important role in the successful treatment of shingles. The valuable mineral proves to be a true all-rounder, for the additional intake of magnesium can alleviate the pain, accelerate the healing process and strengthen nerve and muscle fibers. Therefore, those affected by shingles should pay attention to maintain a nutrition rich in magnesium and vitamins. Of course, the treating physician should be included and consulted in order to determine the ideal dosage.

If you are experiencing chronic pain that has no physical cause, your pain perception may vary substantially. Taking a high dosage of magnesium can result in a noticeable improvement. Basically, it can be used to treat not only shingles, but also migraine, headache, back pain, tumor pain or arthritis. What is especially important with regard to shingles is that magnesium can alleviate neuralgia and nerve damage. In addition, taking magnesium leads to a noticeable relaxation of tense muscles.

Magnesium can block the responsible pain receptors, so that the perceived pain is significantly reduced. This way, strained nerves can be calmed. After taking a high dosage of magnesium, the pain can already be significantly alleviated after around 30 minutes.

Peptidases

Enzymes or proteins are essential for our body, for they fulfill many important tasks. For instance, enzymes are involved in nearly every immune reaction or metabolic reaction. Peptidases are particularly relevant when treating shingles, for they can cleave proteins. The group of peptidases contains among others bromelain, which is extracted from the pineapple plant, and papain, which can be found in papaya. Chymotrypsin and trypsin also belong to the peptidases.

Aside from their anti-inflammatory effect, peptidases also seem to fight viruses in a targeted manner. For instance, a study with 192 participants could determine that an enzyme therapy is just as successful as a therapy with aciclovir, an anti-viral drug, when treating shingles. The participants of the scientific study were divided into two groups. One of these groups was treated according to traditional medical practice, while the other group was treated with an enzyme complex of 400 mg of papain, 160 g of chymotrypsin as well as 160 mg of trypsin. 14 day later, the situation was evaluated, which led to a surprising, but decisive result: In both groups, there were no significant differences in the healing process of the affected individuals. Moreover, it was impressive that there were no side effects in the enzyme therapy, in contrast to the group with the anti-viral drug.

In fact, the treatment with the enzyme cocktail had a positive effect on various bodily functions.

Source: Billigmann: "Enzyme therapy--an alternative in Treatment of Herpes Zoster. A controlled study of 192 Patents".

Shingles can be a very painful and protracted illness. Therefore, many affected individuals also like to draw on alternative remedies such as colloidal silver in additional to their traditional medical treatment. When treating shingles, it can be applied both internally and externally.

Also known as silver water, colloidal silver was frequently used as a natural antibiotic in the past. It played a decisive role in medicine particularly in the 19th century and also at the beginning of the 20th century. It was not until antibiotics were introduced and became widely known that silver water gradually began to disappear. But today, it is experiencing a true renaissance.

Colloidal silver is used quite often in alternative medicine. Especially with infections, it can assist the immune system in successfully fighting the viruses. Additionally, it can also support the regeneration of the skin areas affected by the rash.

Silver water can be drunk to lessen the symptoms of shingles, but it can also be used to treat the inflamed skin areas in a targeted manner. It is advisable to choose a combination of an internal and external application, so the colloidal silver can ideally unfold its effect.

Lysine is a very important amino acid that can cause relief particularly in combatting and containing the pain resulting from shingles. It can be taken as a food supplement in tablet or capsule form, whereby the exact medication should be discussed with the treating physician.

Lysine and especially L-lysine is a proteinogenic and therefore essential amino acid. The reason why it is so important for the human body is that it contributes to strengthening its immune system, among other things. People who have a lysine deficiency often also suffer from an impaired immune system or reduced growth. Taking lysine has a very positive effect on the treatment of shingles. It can cause the pathogens' use of arginine to be reduced and therefore prevent a spreading of the disease, for lysine uses the same transport system as arginine.

If you are supplying your body with arginine when you are suffering from shingles, for instance by consuming cereal products, you should definitely also take lysine in parallel. You can buy corresponding food supplements at a pharmacy or drugstore. It is also advisable to take lysine following shingles because the amino acid promotes the production of collagen and supports the protein structure. This, in turn, benefits the regeneration of the skin. In addition, lysine can improve the skin texture if rough skin areas and skin irritations remain after the characteristic rash.

The amino acid particularly plays an important role in the formation of antibodies and enzymes in the human organism. If you take around one gram of lysine three times a day, it can cause the pain to subside early. The amino acid can have an even stronger effect if you consume little arginine during treatment. Foods such as soy products, nuts, chocolate, oats, seeds and whole grain products contain arginine, which is why those affected should restrict the consumption of these products as far as possible.

As soon as the disease has been overcome, lysine capsules should no longer be taken to prevent an amino acid imbalance. Arginine belongs to the important amino acids, just like lysine. For instance, arginine positively effects the circulation, as it leads to a widening of the blood vessels. But during an infection with the varicella-zoster virus, this positive effect becomes negative, for the viruses use the amino acid to multiply and spread. Therefore, people who have a shingles infection should take little to no arginine, but increase their intake of lysine. Lysine is taken up by the pathogens into their DNA, with the result that the growth is inhibited.

As soon as those affected discover the illness or the first symptoms of shingles, they should make sure to take lysine. Aside from the pure consumption of lysine, it is advisable to also take zinc and vitamin C to achieve an optimum effect. A high dosage of lysine can lead to a constriction of the blood vessels in the long term, which is why you should always consult a doctor regarding your intake of lysine preparations. This particularly applies to all patients who suffer from severe migraine or a cardiovascular disease.

In addition, lysine can support calcium absorption, so taking calcium preparations should be avoided if you are being treated with lysine. If you do not want to take lysine in the form of a food supplement, can also provide your body with the valuable amino acid by changing your diet. As an alternative, you can eat foods such as salmon, pumpkin seeds and chicken breast that are all rich in lysine. Milk, tofu or chicken eggs also contain a lot of lysine. By paying attention to a corresponding and healthy diet, affected individuals can greatly contribute to the successful treatment of shingles themselves. A positive side effect: The amino acid can also reduce the probability of getting recurrent herpes simplex.

The optimum dosage of lysine cannot be generally determined, for it always depends on the respective constitution of the affected individuals and the severity of shingles. Therefore, self-medicating is difficult, which is why the dosage should be determined based on medical consultation.

As a food supplement, lysine in capsule form can be obtained at stationary or online pharmacies, a prescription is normally not required. The average daily requirement is 38 milligrams of L-lysine per kilogram of body weight. The human body can process L-lysine without any problems. Attention: Several preparations often contain a combination of DL-lysine and L-lysine. These food supplements are not as effective in fighting shingles. In addition, an overdose of lysine can entail side effects like blood sugar fluctuations or an impaired blood clotting.

Garlic

Garlic is considered to be very healthy. Consuming garlic can be beneficial for the cardiovascular system and boost your vitality. Additionally, it can also help speed up the healing process when you have shingles. The well-tried and on top of that very reasonably priced home remedy can also prevent infections and alleviate pain.

If you are suffering from an infection with the herpes zoster virus, garlic can ideally be used to alleviate the rash and make it go away more quickly. Simply crush 5 to 6 cloves of garlic and combine them into a paste that is spread on the rash. The paste should remain on the skin for around 15 minutes before it is removed with water. In order to reduce the rash noticeably faster, this treatment should be carried out three times a day.

Propolis tincture

Propolis is a glue used by bees that has an antioxidative and antimicrobial effect. Moreover, it can support the healing process and strengthen the immune system. Individuals who are dealing with shingles can use a propolis tincture to fight the skin rash. For this purpose, the rash is carefully washed with the tincture. This can prevent the secretion of the blisters that have burst open from moving to other skin areas and thus keep the rash from spreading.

Propolis was already used to treat wounds in antiquity and for embalming in ancient Egypt. It can inhibit the growth of pathogens and promote wound healing, for it has an anti-inflammatory effect. In addition, propolis can have a positive impact on the immune system and support the body's defense system.

After treating the rash with the propolis tincture, you can use a propolis salve as an ideal supplement.

St. John's wort

Natural remedies can optimally support the conventional medical treatment of shingles. St. John's wort (Hypericum perforatem) is a herbal sedative and the most famous among the natural remedies. The medicinal plant is closely connected to light.

The shiny yellow blossoms and their impressive filaments resemble small sun wheels. If taken in doses that are too high, St. John's wort can increase our sensitivity to light. The medical herb stands for balance and stability, which can be seen in its straight growth, and can also help us gain more balance and stability.

As a tincture (for example ALCEA or CERES Hypericum), the medicinal plant can brighten your mood and alleviate pain. A so-called mother tincture may only be taken in small quantities, beginning with around one to three drops two to three times a day. Before using a mother tincture, those affected should consult a doctor.

Coneflower (Echinacea purpurea)

Echinacea purpurea, better known as coneflower, can prove to be a useful medicinal plant in the naturopathic treatment of shingles. Therefore, it is advisable to use a tincture that contains coneflower, as it can strengthen the body's defense system. Moreover, coneflower can prevent the dangerous viruses from spreading further. In the acute phase of shingles, the skin rash can additionally be treated with a coneflower tincture in a targeted manner, which can support the healing process. If the rash and blisters subside, this tincture can provide the skin with important nutrients.

Witch hazel

If shingles has already entered its final phase, the blisters have popped and the skin is starting to scab, witch hazel can support wound healing. Aside from wound healing, Hamamelis, as witch hazel is also called by experts, can prevent a bacterial infection as well.

Witch hazel is used in many lotions and ointments. In this form, it can also be used to ideally treat the shingles rash, as it can alleviate the itching sensation. In addition, witch hazel also counteracts inflammation. There is a reason why the indigenous people of North America swore by its healing powers.

Wala oil

If you would like to treat shingles naturally and reduce the pain, you can also use Wala oil. The oil mainly has a pain-relieving effect and is used in particular for neuralgia.

The most important component of this oil is a homeopathic dilution of wolfsbane (aconite). Furthermore, it contains the essential oils of lavender and camphor, which can calm the skin and the nerves.

However, Wala oil should not be used if you have open injuries and infections – meaning that you should avoid using it if the blisters have already popped open. Unless otherwise specified or the package insert states something else, it can be used once or twice a day.

Wala oil can unfold its optimum effect and ease the discomfort resulting from shingles if it is applied directly to the concerned skin areas. For this purpose, massage two or three ml of the oil into the affected areas. Afterwards, the skin should be covered with a wool cloth, so its contents can be directly absorbed by the skin.

Natural yogurt compresses

A very simple and proven household remedy to treat the shingles rash is natural yogurt. For this purpose, the yogurt is placed on the affected areas of the skin in the form of a compress. Natural yogurt compresses can have a very soothing effect on those who are ill with shingles, for they can cool the skin, alleviate the pain and reduce the itching.

Natural yogurt contains several micronutrients that are good for the skin. What is more, yogurt is also very well tolerated, so it can even be used on sensitive skin. It provides the skin with valuable trace elements, minerals and proteins, which can promote the blood circulation and revitalization of the skin. Due to its creamy consistency, it can be easily distributed and is also quickly absorbed.

Natural yogurt compresses can be used both at refrigerator temperature and at room temperature. As an alternative to natural yogurt, you can also use curd.

Chili poultice

The itching can not only be relieved with coldness, but also with warmth, as chili shows. A chili poultice or chili plaster can significantly reduce the itching sensation with warmth and pungency. In addition, this poultice can numb the pain. The muscles are warmed and tensions are relieved. Moreover, it can improve the blood circulation, which can positively affect the body's healing processes.

A chili poultice can be made without much effort. You simply need to take a cloth and dampen it with warm water. In a next step, you sprinkle some chili on it before the chili poultice is placed right on the skin rash. The poultice should stay on the affected part of the body for several minutes. At pharmacies, you can find preparations with chili extract that can naturally also be used for shingles, for instance in the form of lotions.

Alcohol consumption weakens the immune system. Therefore, you should absolutely avoid drinking alcohol if you are suffering from shingles, for it can worsen the progression of the disease. Affected individuals should pay attention to a healthy diet and lifestyle particularly during the disease. As a weakened immune system is considered to be the main cause of shingles, avoiding alcohol can generally also prevent the outbreak of the disease in the first place.

If shingles has broken out, those affected should focus on strengthening their immune system, which can be achieved with a healthy lifestyle. Aside from avoiding alcohol, this also includes making sure to get enough sleep and maintain a high-fiber diet that is rich in vitamins. By the way, not only alcohol, but also nicotine has a negative effect on the circulation. If affected individuals would like the illness do disappear quickly and completely, they should avoid both substances.

Doctors treat shingles with antiviral and pain-relieving medication. Alcohol consumption can have a negative impact on the medical therapy and thus on the healing process, for alcohol can reduce or even change the effectiveness of certain drugs. Interactions and side effects can be the result, which is why consuming alcohol is simply taboo if you have shingles. Coffee is still the most popular drink in Germany, but those affected by the disease should not consume it. For coffee is known to contain caffeine, which gets your circulation going by increasing your heart rate. This, in turn, leads to a deterioration of herpes zoster if you are experiencing shingles. An increased heart rate and excitement immediately impair the immune system, and if it is weakened, a rapid spread of the varicella-zoster viruses is the result. The acute illness can be exacerbated and there can even be a subsequent infection.

Camphor or aconite oil can be used for the external treatment of the skin. The herbal remedies have a pain-relieving effect. Blue rocket (Aconitum napellus) is actually very poisonous. In order to use it as a homeopathic remedy, the plant is gathered with its roots and processed during its blooming time.

It is usually recommended to only use aconite oil during the initial stage of shingles. If puss starts to form and exit the blisters, you should stop using the oil. Only highly diluted homeopathic remedies and ointments that contain aconite are available without prescription. Today, all other types of aconite are only available on prescription because they are difficult to dose.

Aconite oil is a highly effective essential oil that is often also employed to alleviate the symptoms of respiratory diseases and colds. It is used very frequently in creams and lotions. If applied when suffering from a herpes zoster infection, it can not only soothe the pain, but also reduce the rash as well as promote the skin's regeneration and protection due to its microbial qualities.

The herpes zoster viruses are very active and are always trying to multiply and spread. As the bursting blisters are also very infectious, it is advisable to cleanse the skin or the rash with apple vinegar. A spreading can be avoided by carefully cleansing all body areas that are affected by the rash with vinegar water several times a day. At the same time, the vinegar water causes the skin pores to open and the toxins to exit the skin. When cleansing the skin with apple vinegar, the toxins are removed directly. Apple vinegar can also prevent the skin from dehydrating. This is important, as dry skin often cracks. Bacteria can nest in these skin cracks and, in turn, can trigger infections.

Sea buckthorn extract

Vitamin C is particularly important to strengthen the immune system. Aside from an intake through your diet, the body can also be provided with vitamin C from the outside. Sea buckthorn extract is ideal for this purpose, as it has a very high content of vitamin C. The extract can be bought ready for use and all of the affected skin areas can be treated with it directly.

Sea buckthorn extract is won through an extraction of sea buckthorn berries. These berries are very good for the human body, for sea buckthorn is rich in important ingredients such as vitamin C, vitamin B1, vitamin B6 and vitamin B12. Moreover, the berries contain beta-carotene, calcium as well as various elementary minerals. By using sea buckthorn extract, the body can be provided with all of this.

When using the extract, the body's defense mechanisms can be supported tremendously in fighting the viruses. Yet it can not only support the immune system, but also have a regenerating, balancing and pain-relieving effect on the skin that is plagued by the rash.

As an alternative to the extract, you can also use a sea buckthorn paste that can be made from the fresh berries. The paste can cool and calm the skin, which can be perceived to be very soothing. Moreover, sea buckthorn extract can also be taken as a food supplement, whereby it is often administered in capsule form.

(Tormentil, blueberry, common bugle, purple loosestrife)

If you are experiencing acute shingles, your skin is greatly affected by the rash. Lukewarm herbal compresses can accelerate the healing process. The herbs contain many different nutrients that can provide the skin with optimum care and promote the recovery process.

In addition, herbal compresses can also prevent a potential bacterial infection. Tormentil, common bugle, blueberry or also purple loosestrife are particularly suited to treat the shingles rash. Especially the tannins contained in the herbs can positively influence wound healing, for they are anti-inflammatory.

Tormentil in particular has an anti-inflammatory and drying effect, which is especially noticeable in the alleviation of the skin rash. Moreover, it can also inhibit the growth of germs and bacteria.

Blueberries are ideally suited for skin care due to their many antioxidants. The small berries can optimally revitalize the skin, which is especially crucial if you are suffering from strenuous shingles.

The ingredients of common bugle can have a clarifying and purifying effect on the skin. In addition, they support wound healing and alleviate inflammation. Due to its exquisite components and nurturing properties, common bugle is often used in cosmetic products as well.

Purple loosestrife belongs to the barely noticed medicinal plants, although it has a great variety of healing powers. It can support wound healing, alleviate itching, reduce skin inflammations and have an antibacterial effect.

Due to the many special qualities of these medicinal herbs, combining the herbal compresses is an ideal natural remedy for treating shingles.

Clematis recta – better known as the erect clematis – can have a pain-relieving and cooling effect and belongs to the buttercup family. This homeopathic remedy is won from the stems with leaves and blossoms, which are harvested at the beginning of flowering.

Clematis recta can particularly be used against a weeping and itching skin rash – not only if you have shingles. Provided there are no allergies, there are no known side effects to this day. The plant is generally very well tolerated, so children, pregnant or breastfeeding women can also use it. Of course, you should always consult a doctor regarding the intake.

The plant is available in different dosage forms as pills, capsules, drops or globules. The dosage and duration of the treatment depend on the respective preparation, the disease pattern and the severity of the disease.

Charming away shingles with incantations

Charming away different illnesses with incantations is one of the oldest known healing methods. When used against extremely painful shingles, these incantations can often achieve first successes and make the illness subside after only a few days. The earlier these incantations are used, the faster the positive effect can take hold. It is often the case that only a few sessions are necessary, particularly if you begin to charm away shingles at an early stage. This way, the illness can be treated directly in an alternative manner and a strong spread of the viruses can be prevented early on.

Charming away shingles with incantations can generally alleviate all of the typical herpes zoster symptoms. Aside from the actual rose rash, the incantations can also reduce burning skin, itchiness, exhaustion, numbness, sleep disturbances and headaches.

If the herpes zoster infection is still in its acute phase, the rash can subside within a day after the incantations were spoken. No additional rashes begin to form. All of the already existing secretion filled blisters dry up. The pain associated with shingles can already be noticeably alleviated while the incantations are being spoken. If they are spoken in time, the formation of scars or post zoster neuralgia can even be prevented. Charming away shingles with incantations can generally lead to a faster and weakened progression of the illness. Affected individuals who choose to have these incantations used on them often report that even sleep difficulties can disappear as a result.

Of course, those affected by shingles should be receptive towards the incantations and the person performing them. In many cases, alternative practitioners perform these incantations against shingles, but this is not a precondition or a sign of quality. The healer who charms away shingles does not have to be an alternative practitioner.

There are generally no side effects when these incantations are used on shingles. However, it can happen that the symptoms briefly increase after the first or second session before they subside. This is comparable with homeopathy, where it can also be the case that the right remedy temporarily stirs up the symptoms.

The charming process can help those affected relax better. Therefore, it is possible that they temporarily feel particularly tired and their need to sleep increases. Aside from this aspect, however, charming away a herpes zoster infection with incantations is entirely harmless and risk-free.

Trust is essential when incantations are being used against illnesses. Patients need to feel they are in good hands with the healer. If it does not click at an interpersonal level, it is advisable to choose another healer.

Many patients complain they feel tired and at the same time pleasantly exhausted after the first charming session, for the incantations have a calming effect on several people. During the process, affected individuals are freed from their stress and burdens, both of which are factors that often prove to trigger shingles. The strong pain connected to the herpes zoster infection can become an enormous psychological burden. Having shingles charmed away with incantations can prevent this from happening, for body and mind can be healed this way. Those affected have more zest for life and feel a certain drive again – they regain their quality of life.

People who are suffering from shingles and would like to have these incantations used on them do not have to fulfill any special requirements. Their own constitution and general health condition are also not important. However, strong stimuli and extreme stress should be avoided, and the hope for an improvement and healing of the illness should be a constant companion during treatment. Even the smallest successes should be valued. Silent prayers can contribute to the healing process and optimally complement both the charming process and classical therapy.

If painkillers and alternative remedies do not work, it can help to distract yourself when you are experiencing pain. If you engage in a pleasant activity and refocus, you can simply forget the pain.

A good practitioner must have the gift to perform the incantations. However, it is often difficult for laymen to recognize whether a person is truly a gifted healer. But there are several criteria that can be quite revealing. For instance, a healer should be down-to-earth and authentic. He should approach patients, focus on them and give them the feeling they are in good hands with him. While the incantations are being spoken against shingles, the healer exudes a humbleness, calmness and safety and has a calming effect on the patients. In addition, those suffering from the illness should enjoy their sessions with the healer and associate their visit with uplifting feelings. Each session should make them feel positive, so that they look forward to them. By the way, there is no typical incantation performer or healer. If you are looking for someone who can charm away shingles, you should consult your doctor first.

What is the traditional process of charming away shingles with incantations characterized by?

There is no fixed procedure for charming away shingles with incantations. Traditionally, every village had its healer who used these incantations against illnesses. He was normally paid in natural produce. These individuals chose their successor and passed their knowledge on to him – only if he also had the so-called gift, of course. The incantations were not allowed to be spoken, they were strictly confidential.

Today, shingles is charmed away with incantations both in the traditional form and in a modern version. The manner in which they are performed always depends on the healer himself, on his mindset, his knowledge, his gift, his being and his abilities. Affected individuals should always choose their healer carefully. What is decisive for successfully charming away the illness is the patient's belief, but also the connection between the patient and the healer.

I wish you a speedy recovery.